Vitamin D3

A Quick Start Guide for Beginners and a 5-Step Action Plan with an FAQ

mf

copyright © 2024 Patrick Marshwell

All rights reserved No part of this book may be reproduced, or stored in a retrieval system, or transmitted in any form or by any means, electronic, mechanical, photocopying, recording, or otherwise, without express written permission of the publisher.

Disclaimer

By reading this disclaimer, you are accepting the terms of the disclaimer in full. If you disagree with this disclaimer, please do not read the guide.

All of the content within this guide is provided for informational and educational purposes only, and should not be accepted as independent medical or other professional advice. The author is not a doctor, physician, nurse, mental health provider, or registered nutritionist/dietician. Therefore, using and reading this guide does not establish any form of a physician-patient relationship.

Always consult with a physician or another qualified health provider with any issues or questions you might have regarding any sort of medical condition. Do not ever disregard any qualified professional medical advice or delay seeking that advice because of anything you have read in this guide. The information in this guide is not intended to be any sort of medical advice and should not be used in lieu of any medical advice by a licensed and qualified medical professional.

The information in this guide has been compiled from a variety of known sources. However, the author cannot attest to or guarantee the accuracy of each source and thus should not be held liable for any errors or omissions.

You acknowledge that the publisher of this guide will not be held liable for any loss or damage of any kind incurred as a result of this guide or the reliance on any information provided within this guide. You acknowledge and agree that you assume all risk and responsibility for any action you undertake in response to the information in this guide.

Using this guide does not guarantee any particular result (e.g., weight loss or a cure). By reading this guide, you acknowledge that there are no guarantees to any specific outcome or results you can expect.

All product names, diet plans, or names used in this guide are for identification purposes only and are the property of their respective owners. The use of these names does not imply endorsement. All other trademarks cited herein are the property of their respective owners.

Where applicable, this guide is not intended to be a substitute for the original work of this diet plan and is, at most, a supplement to the original work for this diet plan and never a direct substitute. This guide is a personal expression of the facts of that diet plan.

Where applicable, persons shown in the cover images are stock photography models and the publisher has obtained the rights to use the images through license agreements with third-party stock image companies.

Table of Contents

Introduction	6
What Is Vitamin D3?	8
What Is Vitamin D3 Deficiency?	8
Causes of Vitamin D3 Deficiency	9
Symptoms of Vitamin D3 Deficiency	11
Lifestyle Changes to Manage Vitamin D3 Deficiency	13
How Does Vitamin D3 Work?	15
Different Forms of Vitamin D3	18
Use Cases of Vitamin D3 and Health Benefits	22
Health Benefits of Vitamin D3	24
Disadvantages	27
Foods Containing Vitamin D3	30
Natural Sources	30
Fortified Foods	32
5-Step Plan to Start Supplementing Vitamin D3	35
Step 1: Assess Your Current Vitamin D Levels	35
Step 2: Choose the Right Supplement	39
Step 3: Determine the Appropriate Dosage	42
Step 4: Incorporate Vitamin D3 into Your Routine	44
Step 5: Monitor Your Progress and Adjust as Needed	48
Precautions When Taking Vitamin D3 Supplements	52
Potential Side Effects	57
Tips for Maintaining Adequate Vitamin D3 Levels	60
Balancing Sunlight Exposure with Skin Protection	60
Incorporating Vitamin D3-rich Foods into the Diet	67
Choosing and Using Supplements Correctly	69
Conclusion	73
FAQs	77
References and Helpful Links	80

Introduction

Have you ever stopped to think about how crucial Vitamin D3 is to your daily health? Known as the "sunshine vitamin," Vitamin D3 is more than just a nutrient; it's a silent contributor to overall well-being that is often overlooked. As our lives become increasingly occupied with indoor activities and diligent sun protection, many people unknowingly suffer from a deficiency in this essential vitamin. This growing concern raises an important question: Are we getting enough Vitamin D3 to support our health?

In today's fast-paced world, the relevance of Vitamin D3 cannot be understated. Our modern lifestyle choices have significantly reduced our natural exposure to sunlight, which is the primary source of Vitamin D3. With less time spent outdoors, many people are not meeting their daily Vitamin D3 needs, leading to a widespread deficiency that often goes unnoticed. Understanding this gap is vital as it highlights the importance of being proactive about our health.

Addressing Vitamin D3 deficiency doesn't have to be a daunting task. By incorporating a high-quality Vitamin D3 supplement into your daily routine, you can take a simple yet effective step towards ensuring your body receives the nutrients it requires. Whether through supplements, dietary changes, or safe sun exposure, there are multiple ways to bridge the gap and enhance your health.

In this guide, you will learn about the following:

- What is Vitamin D3?
- What is Vitamin D3 Deficiency?
- How does Vitamin D3 work?
- Use Cases and Health Benefits of Vitamin D3
- Step-Guide on How to Get Started in Supplementing Vitamin D3
- Foods Containing Vitamin D3

Keep reading to discover how you can effortlessly incorporate Vitamin D3 into your daily routine. By exploring a variety of supplement options, you can find the perfect fit for your lifestyle, ensuring that you meet your health needs seamlessly. At the end of this guide, you'll have a better understanding of why Vitamin D3 is essential and how it can positively impact your overall well-being.

What Is Vitamin D3?

Vitamin D3, is a type of vitamin D that is produced in the skin in response to sunlight exposure. It is also found in some foods and can be taken as a dietary supplement.

Vitamin D3 is essential for bone health as it facilitates the absorption of calcium & phosphorus in the body. It aids immune system function and is associated with mood stabilization and general well-being. Deficiency in vitamin D3 can lead to bone disorders such as rickets in children and osteomalacia in adults.

What Is Vitamin D3 Deficiency?

Vitamin D3 deficiency occurs when there is an insufficient level of Vitamin D3 in the body. This can lead to a range of health issues because Vitamin D3 plays a crucial role in numerous bodily functions such as absorbing calcium, maintaining bone health, and supporting the body's immune system.

If left untreated, it can lead to more severe conditions like osteoporosis in adults or rickets in children. It's important to address any deficiency with dietary changes, supplements, or increased sun exposure, ideally under the guidance of a medical expert.

Causes of Vitamin D3 Deficiency

Vitamin D3 deficiency can be caused by several factors, including:

1. *Limited Sun Exposure*: Spending too much time indoors, particularly in our increasingly digital world, can significantly hinder our skin's ability to synthesize Vitamin D3 from sunlight. Living in areas with prolonged winters or using sunscreen excessively can worsen the situation. Although sunscreen protects against harmful UV rays, it can also hinder the sunlight required for Vitamin D synthesis.

2. *Geographic Location*: Those who reside in higher latitudes experience less direct sunlight, especially during the winter months when days are shorter. This reduced exposure can lead to a notable decrease in Vitamin D3 production, making it essential for individuals in these areas to find alternative sources of this vital nutrient.

3. *Skin Pigmentation*: Individuals with darker skin tones possess higher levels of melanin, which can act as a natural barrier to UV radiation. While this provides

certain protective benefits against skin damage, it can also limit the skin's ability to effectively produce Vitamin D3 from sunlight, making supplementation or dietary sources more important for these individuals.

4. *Age*: As people grow older, various physiological changes occur that impede the skin's ability to synthesize Vitamin D3. These changes include a decrease in the skin's thickness and its overall efficiency in converting sunlight into Vitamin D3. Additionally, the kidneys become less efficient at transforming Vitamin D3 into its active form, further compounding the issue for older adults.

5. *Dietary Intake*: A well-balanced diet is crucial for maintaining adequate levels of Vitamin D3. Those who do not consume enough foods rich in this vitamin, such as fatty fish, fortified dairy products, and egg yolks, may find themselves at risk of deficiency. It is vital to incorporate these nutrient-dense foods into one's diet to support overall health and well-being.

6. *Medical Conditions*: Certain health conditions can significantly interfere with the body's ability to absorb Vitamin D3 effectively. For instance, diseases like Crohn's disease, celiac disease, and cystic fibrosis can disrupt intestinal absorption, leading to lower levels of this essential vitamin. Individuals with these

conditions should consult healthcare providers for tailored guidance on managing their Vitamin D levels.

7. ***Obesity***: Vitamin D3 is a fat-soluble vitamin, which means it can be stored in body fat. Individuals with higher body fat percentages may have lower circulating levels of Vitamin D3 because the vitamin gets sequestered in fat tissues, making it less available for use by the body. This dynamic highlights the importance of monitoring Vitamin D levels in individuals with obesity and may necessitate adjusted dietary or supplementation strategies.

These factors can contribute to insufficient Vitamin D3 levels, impacting overall health and well-being.

Symptoms of Vitamin D3 Deficiency

Symptoms of Vitamin D3 deficiency can vary significantly among individuals, but there are several common signs that you should be aware of:

1. ***Fatigue and Tiredness***: Persistent low energy levels and an unusual sense of fatigue can be early indicators of Vitamin D3 deficiency. This fatigue may not improve with rest, making daily activities feel more challenging.

2. ***Bone Pain and Weakness***: Vitamin D3 plays a crucial role in maintaining bone health by helping the body

absorb calcium. A deficiency can lead to bone pain, tenderness, or a general feeling of weakness in the muscles, potentially impacting mobility and daily function.

3. *Frequent Infections*: A weakened immune system due to low Vitamin D3 levels may make you more susceptible to infections. Individuals with a deficiency often experience more frequent colds, flu, or other infections, indicating that their bodies struggle to fight off illnesses.

4. *Mood Changes*: Research has linked Vitamin D3 deficiency to mood disorders, including depression and anxiety. Low levels of this vitamin can affect the production of mood-regulating neurotransmitters, leading to emotional imbalances that can affect overall quality of life.

5. *Slow Wound Healing*: Cuts, bruises, and other injuries may take longer to heal if your Vitamin D3 levels are insufficient. This can be concerning, particularly for individuals who have underlying health conditions that already impair healing.

6. *Hair Loss*: Severe Vitamin D3 deficiency can contribute to hair loss, particularly in women. This can manifest as thinning hair or an increase in shedding, which can be distressing and impact self-esteem.

7. *Muscle Pain*: Unexplained muscle pain or cramps can sometimes be a symptom of low Vitamin D3 levels. This discomfort may be more pronounced after physical activity or during periods of inactivity, leading to a cycle of avoidance and further weakness.

8. *Bone Loss*: Over time, a deficiency in Vitamin D3 can lead to decreased bone density, which increases the risk of fractures and osteoporosis. This is particularly concerning for older adults, as maintaining bone strength is vital for preventing falls and related injuries.

If you suspect you are experiencing symptoms of Vitamin D3 deficiency, it is crucial to consult a healthcare provider. They can perform proper testing to assess your Vitamin D levels and provide guidance on how to address any deficiencies through diet, supplements, or lifestyle changes.

Lifestyle Changes to Manage Vitamin D3 Deficiency

Managing Vitamin D3 deficiency can be effectively achieved through simple lifestyle modifications. Here are some practical strategies to help boost your Vitamin D3 levels and improve your overall health:

1. *Increase Sun Exposure*: Try to spend more time outdoors, especially during midday when the sun is at

its peak. Aim for 10-30 minutes of direct sunlight several times a week, depending on your skin type and sensitivity. Remember, just a little sun exposure can significantly enhance Vitamin D3 production.

2. ***Dietary Adjustments***: Incorporate foods rich in Vitamin D3 into your diet. Fatty fish like salmon, mackerel, and tuna are excellent sources. Additionally, include fortified dairy products, egg yolks, and liver to increase your intake.

3. ***Regular Exercise***: Engage in regular physical activity to support bone health and improve overall well-being. Weight-bearing exercises, such as walking, jogging, and resistance training, are particularly beneficial for strengthening bones and enhancing Vitamin D3 metabolism.

4. ***Consider Supplements***: If lifestyle changes alone aren't sufficient, Vitamin D supplements may be an option. It's important to consult with a healthcare provider to determine the appropriate dosage and ensure it aligns with your health needs.

By adopting these lifestyle changes, you can effectively manage Vitamin D3 deficiency and support your body's health. Embrace these steps with a positive mindset, and you'll be on your way to maintaining adequate Vitamin D3 levels.

How Does Vitamin D3 Work?

Vitamin D3 works by helping the body absorb calcium & phosphorus, these are crucial for developing and preserving strong bones and teeth.. Here's a breakdown of how it functions:

1. **Synthesis and Activation**

    When your skin is bare, particularly the UVB rays, it initiates a crucial process that synthesizes vitamin D3, which is essential for various bodily functions. This is then transported to the liver, where it undergoes a conversion process into calcidiol, a form that can be stored in the body.

    In the kidneys, calcidiol is subsequently converted into calcitriol, the active vitamin D form crucial for regulating blood levels of calcium & phosphorus.. promoting healthy bone development, and supporting immune function. This intricate process underscores the importance of sunlight for our overall health.

2. **Calcium and Phosphorus Regulation**

   As the active form of vitamin D, calcitriol is essential for improving the uptake of calcium & phosphorus from the digestive tract into the blood. This process is vital because calcium & phosphorus are key minerals necessary for various bodily functions, particularly for the health of our bones and teeth. By facilitating the uptake of these minerals, calcitriol ensures that they are readily available in the blood for critical physiological processes.

   Additionally, calcitriol maintains the proper balance of calcium and phosphorus, preventing deficiencies that could lead to bone disorders such as rickets in children or osteomalacia in adults. This regulatory process is crucial for supporting ideal bone development and upkeep throughout life, emphasizing the significance of sufficient vitamin D levels for overall bone health.

3. **Bone Health**

   Vitamin D3 plays a crucial role in promoting calcium absorption in the body, which is vital for maintaining proper bone density and strength. This essential nutrient aids in the regulation of calcium & phosphorus levels, ensuring that bones remain strong and resilient.

By supporting these processes, vitamin D3 significantly reduces the risk of fractures and bone-related diseases, such as osteoporosis. Ensuring adequate vitamin D3 intake, whether through sunlight exposure, dietary sources, or supplements, is essential for overall bone health and longevity.

4. **Immune System Support**

Vitamin D3 is vital for adjusting the immune system by encouraging the creation of antimicrobial peptides, which assist in fighting infections. It boosts the body's defense capabilities, enhancing its efficiency in recognizing and responding to pathogens.

By ensuring adequate levels of Vitamin D3, individuals may strengthen their immune response, potentially reducing the risk of illnesses and supporting overall health.

5. **Other Functions**

In addition to its primary roles, it may also play a significant role in influencing cell growth, and promoting healthy cellular development and regeneration. Furthermore, it can impact neuromuscular function by enhancing communication between nerves and muscles, leading to improved coordination and strength.

It is also known for its potential to reduce inflammation, which can help alleviate pain and support overall health by minimizing the body's inflammatory response to injury or stress.

Vitamin D3 is vital for maintaining various bodily functions, particularly those related to bone health and immune support.

Different Forms of Vitamin D3

Vitamin D3 is available in several forms, primarily distinguished by how they are consumed or administered. Here are the different forms:

1. **Capsules/Tablets**

   These are the most prevalent types of vitamin D3 supplements, readily accessible in a range of dosages to meet diverse daily intake requirements. They provide an easy method to maintain sufficient vitamin D levels, which are crucial for bone health, immune support, and general well-being.

   Many manufacturers provide coated options to enhance swallowing ease, and it's important to follow recommended dosages to achieve optimal benefits.

2. **Softgels**

   These are similar to capsules in that they both serve as a convenient way to deliver supplements or medications. However, soft gels typically feature a gelatinous coating that makes them easier to swallow, especially for those who may have difficulty with traditional hard capsules.

This coating also allows for faster dissolution in the stomach, which can enhance the absorption of the active ingredients. Softgels are often preferred for their smooth texture and the ability to encapsulate oils and liquid formulations effectively.

3. **Liquid Drops**

These are an excellent option for individuals who have trouble swallowing pills or require precise dosage adjustments. Liquid drops offer the flexibility to easily modify the amount taken based on specific needs, making them ideal for both adults and children.

Additionally, they can be seamlessly added to food or beverages, ensuring that taking medication becomes a more convenient and pleasant experience. This method not only enhances ease of consumption but also allows for better absorption of the active ingredients into the body.

4. **Gummies**

These chewable supplements come in a variety of flavors, making them a fun and tasty option for both children and adults who may find it difficult to swallow traditional pills. Their appealing texture and sweetness not only enhance the experience of taking vitamins or supplements but also help encourage consistent usage, as many people enjoy the process of chewing them.

Whether they're packed with essential vitamins, minerals, or other health-boosting ingredients, gummies have become a popular choice for anyone looking to maintain their wellness in a more enjoyable way.

5. Powder

This versatile option can be easily mixed with water, juice, or other beverages, providing a convenient alternative for those who prefer not to take pills or gummies. Powders can come in various flavors, making them easier to incorporate into your daily routine. Additionally, they often dissolve quickly, allowing for seamless consumption on the go, perfect for busy lifestyles.

6. Fortified Foods

Certain foods, like milk, orange juice, and breakfast cereals, are frequently enriched with vitamin D3. This involves incorporating vitamin D3 into these items to boost their nutritional content, making them a great dietary option for those who might not get enough sunlight. Including fortified foods in your diet can help maintain sufficient vitamin D levels, which are vital for bone health and overall wellness.

7. **Injections**

    In certain medical situations, vitamin D3 can be administered through injections, a method often employed when a rapid correction of deficiency is necessary. This approach is particularly useful for individuals who may have difficulty absorbing vitamin D through oral supplements due to gastrointestinal issues or those with severely low levels.

    Typically, these injections are given under the careful supervision of a healthcare professional, who can monitor the patient's response and adjust dosage as needed to ensure optimal results and minimize any potential side effects.

These forms cater to different preferences and needs, making it easier for individuals to incorporate vitamin D3 into their daily routines.

Use Cases of Vitamin D3 and Health Benefits

Vitamin D3 is a versatile nutrient with a range of health benefits that extend across various bodily systems. The following are the most common use cases of Vitamin D3:

1. **Preventing and Managing Osteoporosis**

    Vitamin D3 plays a crucial role in bone health by enhancing the absorption of calcium & phosphorus, essential minerals for bone formation and maintenance. This makes it vital for preventing osteoporosis, a condition characterized by weak and brittle bones.

    Studies have shown that adequate levels of Vitamin D3 can help increase bone density and reduce the risk of fractures in older adults, turning it into a critical component of osteoporosis management strategies.

2. **Supporting Immune Health During Cold Seasons**

    Vitamin D3 is known to bolster the body's immune system, which is especially beneficial during cold and flu seasons. It helps modulate the immune response by activating T cells, which are crucial for fighting off pathogens. Research suggests that individuals with higher levels of Vitamin D3 are less likely to catch colds and other respiratory infections, highlighting its importance in maintaining immune resilience.

3. Enhancing Athletic Performance and Recovery

Athletes can benefit from Vitamin D3's role in muscle function and recovery. It aids in muscle strength by promoting protein synthesis and reducing inflammation following intense physical activity.

Additionally, Vitamin D3 supports cardiovascular health, which can enhance endurance and performance. Supplementing with Vitamin D3 has been associated with improved physical performance and faster recovery times, turning it into a valuable nutrient for athletes.

4. Managing Autoimmune Disorders

Vitamin D3 has been linked to the management of autoimmune disorders, conditions where the body's immune system attacks the body's tissues. It acts as an immunomodulator, helping to regulate immune function and reduce inflammatory responses that are often present in autoimmune conditions like multiple sclerosis, rheumatoid arthritis, and lupus. Emerging research indicates that adequate Vitamin D3 levels may help reduce the severity and frequency of autoimmune flare-ups.

5. **Potential Role in Mental Health Treatments**

Recent studies have explored the connection between Vitamin D3 and mental health, suggesting that it may play a role in mood regulation and cognitive function. Deficiency in Vitamin D3 has been associated with an increased risk of depression and other mood disorders.

Some research indicates that supplementation can improve symptoms of depression and anxiety, potentially by influencing the production of neurotransmitters and reducing inflammation in the brain.

Overall, Vitamin D3 is a critical nutrient with diverse applications in health and wellness. Its ability to support bone health, enhance immune function, and potentially influence mental well-being makes it an important consideration for both preventive and therapeutic health strategies.

Health Benefits of Vitamin D3

Vitamin D3 is a vital nutrient with numerous health benefits that impact various aspects of human health. Here's an in-depth exploration of its essential functions:

1. **Role in Calcium Absorption and Bone Health:**

   Vitamin D3 is vital for bone health as it aids in the absorption of calcium. It helps the intestines absorb calcium from the diet, which is necessary for building and maintaining strong bones.

   Without sufficient Vitamin D3, the body cannot absorb adequate amounts of calcium, leading to weakened bones and conditions such as osteoporosis. Studies have shown that adequate Vitamin D3 levels can help prevent fractures and maintain bone density, particularly in older adults.

2. **Immune System Support**

   Vitamin D3 is known for its immune-boosting properties. It helps regulate the body's immune system, ensuring a balanced response to pathogens. Vitamin D3 activates immune cells, such as T cells, which play a critical role in identifying and attacking foreign invaders like bacteria and viruses.

   Research indicates that individuals with higher levels of Vitamin D3 are less susceptible to infections, particularly respiratory infections, turning it into an important nutrient for immune health, especially during cold and flu seasons.

3. **Influence on Mood and Mental Health**

   Vitamin D3 has been linked to mood regulation and mental health. It influences the production of neurotransmitters, which are chemicals in the brain that affect mood and cognitive function. Deficiency in Vitamin D3 has been associated with an increased risk of depression and anxiety.

   Some studies suggest that Vitamin D3 supplementation can improve symptoms of depression by supporting brain health and reducing inflammation. This connection highlights its potential role in mental health treatments.

4. **Importance for Muscle Function**

   Vitamin D3 is essential for optimal muscle function. It contributes to muscle strength by supporting protein synthesis and reducing muscle inflammation, particularly after exercise. This is important for maintaining mobility and reducing the risk of falls in older adults. Athletes also benefit from Vitamin D3, as it aids in muscle recovery and performance, turning it into a valuable component of fitness and rehabilitation programs.

5. **Potential Roles in Disease Prevention**

   Emerging research suggests that Vitamin D3 may play a role in preventing certain diseases, including heart disease, diabetes, and cancer. It is believed to have anti-inflammatory and immune-modulating effects that could help reduce the risk of chronic diseases. For heart health, Vitamin D3 may help control blood pressure and improve arterial function.

In diabetes, it may improve insulin sensitivity and glucose metabolism. Additionally, some studies indicate that adequate Vitamin D3 levels may reduce the risk of certain cancers by promoting healthy cell growth and reducing inflammation.

Vitamin D3 is a multifaceted nutrient with significant health benefits, turning it into an essential part of maintaining overall health and preventing various conditions. Ensuring adequate intake through sunlight exposure, diet, or supplementation can help harness these benefits effectively.

Disadvantages

While Vitamin D3 is essential for numerous bodily functions and overall health, it's important to acknowledge certain disadvantages that could arise, primarily due to excessive intake or improper management. However, it is crucial to note that the benefits of Vitamin D3 significantly outweigh these potential drawbacks when managed properly.

1. **Potential Side Effects of Excessive Intake**

   One of the primary concerns with Vitamin D3 is hypercalcemia, a condition characterized by elevated calcium levels in the blood. Hypercalcemia can lead to a range of health issues, including nausea, vomiting, weakness, and in severe cases, kidney damage. This condition is typically the result of consuming Vitamin D3 in excessive amounts, often through overuse of supplements, rather than through diet or sunlight alone.

2. **Interactions with Medications**

   Vitamin D3 may interact with certain medications, which could affect their efficacy or lead to adverse effects. For instance, it can alter the way the body processes medications like steroids, weight-loss drugs, or cholesterol-lowering medications. It's always recommended to consult with a healthcare provider before starting any new supplement regimen to ensure it won't interfere with existing medications.

3. **Risk of Skin Damage**

   For those seeking to boost their Vitamin D3 levels through sun exposure, there is a risk of skin damage, including sunburn, and an increased risk of skin cancer, due to prolonged exposure to UV rays. It's important to balance sun exposure with skin protection measures, such as using sunscreen or wearing protective clothing, to minimize these risks.

Despite these disadvantages, the benefits of maintaining adequate Vitamin D3 levels are substantial. It supports bone health, enhances immune function, aids in mood regulation, and contributes to muscle strength, among other benefits. By monitoring intake and being mindful of sun exposure, individuals can enjoy the numerous health advantages of Vitamin D3 while minimizing potential drawbacks.

Foods Containing Vitamin D3

Vitamin D3, also known as cholecalciferol, can be found in a variety of foods, both natural and fortified. Here's a list of foods rich in Vitamin D3:

Natural Sources

1. **Fatty Fish**
    - *Salmon:* Considered one of the best natural sources of Vitamin D3, salmon offers a wealth of health benefits. This fatty fish isn't only rich in omega-3 fatty acids, which are essential for heart and brain health, but it also contains high-quality protein, vitamins, and minerals. Including salmon in the foods you eat might help reduce inflammation, improve cognitive function, and support overall well-being. Whether grilled, baked, or enjoyed in sushi, salmon is a delicious way to nourish your body.
    - *Mackerel:* This nutritious fish is not only packed with Vitamin D3, which is essential for maintaining healthy bones and immune

function, but it also provides a substantial amount of protein and healthy omega-3 fatty acids. These beneficial fats are known to support heart health and brain function, making mackerel an excellent choice for those looking to enhance their diet with nutrient-rich options. Additionally, its rich flavor makes it a versatile ingredient in various dishes.

2. **Cod Liver Oil**

   Renowned for its high Vitamin D3 content, cod liver oil is derived from the liver of cod fish and is an excellent source of essential nutrients. In addition to being rich in omega-3 fatty acids, which play a crucial role in heart health and reducing inflammation, it also contains Vitamin A, vital for maintaining healthy vision, supporting immune function, and promoting skin health.

   Regular consumption of cod liver oil can contribute to overall well-being, turning it into a valuable addition to a balanced diet.

3. **Egg Yolks**

   Egg yolks are a rich source of nutrition, containing moderate amounts of Vitamin D3, which is essential for bone health and immune function. In addition to Vitamin D3, they also provide a variety of other nutrients, including high-quality protein that supports muscle repair and growth, B vitamins that play a crucial role in energy metabolism, and essential fats that are important for overall health. Incorporating egg yolks into the foods you eat might contribute to a balanced nutrition plan while offering a delicious and versatile ingredient for various dishes.

Fortified Foods

1. Fortified Milk and Dairy Products

Cow's milk is frequently fortified with Vitamin D3, which enhances its nutritional profile and makes it a convenient source of this essential vitamin for those who regularly consume dairy. This fortification is especially beneficial for individuals who may not get enough sunlight, as Vitamin D3 plays an essential role in the body's ability to absorb calcium.

Besides Vitamin D3, cow's milk contains a substantial amount of calcium, a mineral that collaborates with Vitamin D3 to support the development of strong and healthy bones. Incorporating fortified dairy products into the foods you eat might help ensure you meet your nutritional needs, particularly for bone health, turning it into a smart choice for individuals of all ages, from children to the elderly.

2. **Breakfast Cereals**

   Many breakfast cereals are fortified with Vitamin D3, providing a convenient and effective method to enhance your daily intake of this essential nutrient. When consumed with milk, which also contains calcium and other important vitamins, these cereals create a healthy beginning to your morning.

   This combination not only supports healthy bones and immune function but also makes breakfast a simple yet powerful meal choice for busy individuals and families looking to enhance their overall well-being.

3. **Plant-Based Milk Alternatives**

   Soy, almond, and oat milk are increasingly popular choices among consumers seeking non-dairy options. These alternatives are often fortified with Vitamin D3, which is essential for bone health and immune function, making them suitable substitutes for traditional dairy milk, especially for those following a plant-based diet.

   In addition to Vitamin D3, many brands enhance their formulations with additional nutrients such as calcium, which supports bone density, and vitamins B12 and E, both of which play vital roles in overall health. This fortification helps ensure that individuals who choose plant-based milk can still meet their nutritional needs while enjoying a variety of flavors and textures.

These foods offer a range of options to help meet your Vitamin D3 needs, supporting overall health and wellness.

5-Step Plan to Start Supplementing Vitamin D3

Vitamin D3, commonly known as the "sunshine vitamin," is vital for maintaining good health. It is important for bone health, aids immune system function, and is associated with mood regulation. Despite its importance, many people find it challenging to obtain sufficient Vitamin D3 from sunlight and diet alone. Taking Vitamin D3 supplements can help fill this gap and promote overall wellness.

Step 1: Assess Your Current Vitamin D Levels

Before embarking on any Vitamin D supplementation regimen, it is crucial to first assess your current Vitamin D levels. This preliminary step ensures a tailored approach to your health needs, preventing potential health risks associated with improper supplementation.

Why Knowing Your Vitamin D Levels is Essential

Vitamin D is crucial in various bodily functions, including bone health, immune function, and inflammation regulation.

This vital nutrient facilitates the uptake of calcium & phosphorus, which are crucial for maintaining strong bones and teeth.

Additionally, adequate levels of Vitamin D support the body's immune system by boosting the infection-fighting abilities of monocytes and macrophages—white blood cells essential for our immune defense. Research has also suggested that Vitamin D may help prevent chronic diseases such as diabetes, heart disease, and certain cancers by influencing cellular growth and immune responses.

However, it's important to recognize that both deficiency and excess of Vitamin D can lead to health problems. A deficiency that can lead to weakened bones, heightening the risk of fractures and diseases such as osteoporosis, while excessive Vitamin D can lead to toxicity, potentially causing symptoms such as nausea, weakness, and kidney damage.

Given these implications, it is essential to know your Vitamin D levels before starting any supplements or making significant dietary changes, ensuring that you maintain optimal health and well-being. Regular testing can help you monitor your levels and adjust your intake accordingly.

How to Schedule a Blood Test
Assessing your Vitamin D levels is an important step in maintaining your overall health, and scheduling a blood test with your healthcare provider is a straightforward process.

Start by contacting your doctor's office to set up an appointment; be prepared to discuss your health history and any specific symptoms you may be experiencing that could warrant testing. Alternatively, you can visit a local clinic or lab that offers vitamin testing services, which may provide more flexible scheduling options.

When you arrive for your appointment, a healthcare professional will guide you through the process. They will take a small blood sample, typically from a vein in your arm, using a sterile needle. This procedure is quick and usually takes just a few minutes. After your blood is drawn, it will be sent to a laboratory for analysis, where it will be tested to determine your Vitamin D status.

Depending on the clinic or lab, you may be able to receive your results through a patient portal or during a follow-up consultation with your healthcare provider. It's essential to follow up on your results and discuss any necessary lifestyle changes or supplementation options to ensure your Vitamin D levels remain optimal.

Interpreting Your Blood Test Results

Once your blood test results are available, your healthcare provider will schedule a consultation to discuss them with you in detail. This conversation is an important opportunity to understand what the results mean for your health and to address any questions or concerns you may have. Vitamin D levels are typically measured in nanograms per milliliter (ng/mL), which is a standard unit of measurement in medical laboratories.

In general, a Vitamin D level ranging from 20 ng/mL to 50 ng/mL is considered adequate for healthy individuals, indicating that your body is receiving enough of this vital nutrient to support bone health, immune function, and overall wellness. However, levels below 20 ng/mL are a cause for concern and indicate a deficiency, which may lead to issues such as weakened bones, increased susceptibility to infections, and other health complications.

Conversely, levels above 50 ng/mL might suggest excessive Vitamin D intake, often due to over-supplementation, which can be detrimental to your health. Too much Vitamin D can cause hypercalcemia, a condition marked by increased calcium levels in the bloodstream—which may cause nausea, weakness, and serious complications if not addressed. It's important to monitor your Vitamin D levels regularly and consult with your healthcare provider to ensure they remain within the optimal range for your health needs.

Potential Risks of Over-Supplementation

While Vitamin D is vital for health, over-supplementation can lead to toxicity. Symptoms of Vitamin D toxicity include nausea, vomiting, weakness, and serious complications like kidney damage. By knowing your Vitamin D levels, you can avoid these risks by taking supplements in appropriate doses as recommended by your healthcare provider.

Understanding your Vitamin D levels before starting a supplement regimen is a critical step in ensuring optimal health and preventing the adverse effects of over-supplementation. By scheduling a blood test and consulting with your healthcare provider, you can make informed decisions about your Vitamin D intake and maintain a balanced approach to your health.

Step 2: Choose the Right Supplement

After determining your Vitamin D levels, the next crucial step is selecting the right supplement to meet your needs. This decision should be guided by your test results and the quality of the supplement you choose, ensuring you gain the maximum benefit from your regimen.

Understanding Vitamin D3 vs. Vitamin D2

Vitamin D supplements come in two primary forms: Vitamin D3 (cholecalciferol) and Vitamin D2 (ergocalciferol). Vitamin D3 is derived from animal sources, such as fish liver oil and egg yolks, and is the same form of your body naturally produces Vitamin D when exposed to sunlight.. This conversion occurs in the skin when ultraviolet B (UVB) rays hit it, allowing for optimal absorption and utilization by the body.

In contrast, Vitamin D2 is plant-based, often sourced from yeast and mushrooms exposed to UV light. While both forms can help increase Vitamin D levels, research has shown that Vitamin D3 is generally more effective at raising and maintaining adequate Vitamin D levels in the blood compared to D2.

This is primarily due to Vitamin D3's superior bioavailability and longer half-life in the body, making it the preferred choice for most individuals seeking to optimize their Vitamin D status for improved bone health, immune function, and overall well-being. Consequently, many healthcare professionals recommend Vitamin D3 supplements for those looking to boost their intake.

Why Vitamin D3 Is Often Preferred

The preference for Vitamin D3 over D2 is primarily attributed to its superior ability to elevate serum concentrations of Vitamin D in the body. Research studies have shown that Vitamin D3, also known as cholecalciferol, remains in the bloodstream for a longer duration compared to its counterpart, D2 (ergocalciferol). This extended presence in the blood translates to more effective utilization by the body.

Additionally, Vitamin D3 is more effective at converting into calcitriol, the active form of Vitamin D, which is vital for controlling calcium and phosphate levels, thereby promoting bone strength and enhancing immune function. Its enhanced potency makes Vitamin D3 a more reliable option for correcting deficiencies and maintaining optimal health, particularly in individuals who may be at risk of insufficiency due to limited sun exposure or dietary intake.

Additionally, many healthcare professionals recommend D3 supplements for their effectiveness in promoting overall wellness and preventing chronic diseases linked to low Vitamin D levels.

Identifying High-Quality Supplements

When choosing a Vitamin D3 supplement, it is vital to focus on quality to ensure you are getting the most effective product for your health. Look for supplements that are sourced from reputable manufacturers known for their rigorous quality control standards, as this can significantly impact the potency and safety of the supplement. Investigate the company's background, checking for certifications and third-party testing, which can provide additional assurance of the product's purity and efficacy.

Opt for products with clear labeling that not only indicates the source of Vitamin D3—whether it is derived from fish liver oil, lichen, or synthetic sources—but also specifies the dosage per serving to help you make informed decisions based on your individual health needs.

Furthermore, it's important to choose supplements that are free from unnecessary fillers, binders, or artificial additives, as these can detract from the overall quality and effectiveness of the supplement. By taking these factors into account, you can ensure you select a high-quality Vitamin D3 supplement that supports your overall well-being.

The Importance of Third-Party Testing

Third-party testing is a crucial factor in assessing the quality of a Vitamin D supplement. Supplements that have been third-party tested undergo evaluation by independent organizations to verify their purity, potency, and safety. This certification ensures that the product contains the ingredients listed on the label in the correct amounts and is free from contaminants. Check for logos from organizations such as NSF International, ConsumerLab, or the U.S. Pharmacopeia (USP) on the package.

Selecting the right Vitamin D supplement involves understanding the differences between Vitamin D3 and D2, prioritizing high-quality products, and ensuring third-party testing. By taking these steps, you can confidently choose a supplement that effectively supports your health needs and contributes to maintaining adequate Vitamin D levels.

Step 3: Determine the Appropriate Dosage

Once you've identified the right Vitamin D supplement, the next essential step involves determining the appropriate dosage. This ensures you receive the optimal amount needed for your health without risking potential side effects.

Factors Influencing Dosage Needs

Several factors can influence your Vitamin D3 dosage needs, including age, body weight, geographic location, lifestyle, dietary habits, and underlying health conditions. For instance, individuals living in areas with limited sunlight exposure, those with darker skin, or people who spend most of their time indoors may require higher dosages.

Additionally, certain medical conditions or medications can impact Vitamin D metabolism, necessitating adjustments in supplementation.

The Role of Healthcare Providers

Consulting with a healthcare provider is critical when determining your Vitamin D3 dosage. A healthcare professional can assess your personal health status, review your blood test results, and consider any specific health needs you might have. They can also monitor your progress and make dosage adjustments as necessary, ensuring your Vitamin D levels remain within a safe and effective range.

General Dosage Guidelines for Adults

While personalized recommendations are ideal, general guidelines suggest that adults typically require between 600 to 2000 International Units (IU) of Vitamin D3 per day. The lower end of this range is often recommended for maintaining general health, while higher dosages may be necessary for addressing deficiencies. It's important to note that these are broad recommendations, and individual needs can vary significantly.

Importance of Personalized Dosage Plans

A personalized dosage plan is essential for optimizing Vitamin D3 supplementation. By tailoring the dosage to your specific needs, you can prevent both deficiency and over-supplementation, reducing the risk of adverse effects like Vitamin D toxicity. Personalized plans also allow for adjustments based on changes in lifestyle, health status, or seasonal variations in sunlight exposure.

Determining the appropriate dosage of Vitamin D3 involves considering various personal factors and consulting with healthcare professionals for tailored guidance. By understanding your unique needs and following expert recommendations, you can effectively manage your Vitamin D levels and support overall well-being.

Step 4: Incorporate Vitamin D3 into Your Routine

Successfully incorporating Vitamin D3 into your daily routine is essential for reaping its full health benefits. Ensuring consistency in taking your supplement can help maintain optimal Vitamin D levels, supporting bone health, immune function, and overall well-being.

Choosing the Best Time for Supplementation

Selecting a specific time of day to take your Vitamin D3 supplement can greatly enhance your ability to remember it consistently. While there is no definitive time that is universally best, integrating it into a routine activity can serve as a helpful reminder.

Some people prefer taking their supplements in the morning as part of their breakfast routine, while others might find it more convenient during lunch or dinner.

Benefits of Taking Vitamin D3 with Meals

Vitamin D is a fat-soluble nutrient, which means it is most effectively absorbed when consumed with dietary fats. Taking your Vitamin D3 supplement with a meal that includes healthy fats can significantly improve its absorption.

Foods like avocados, nuts, seeds, olive oil, and fatty fish are excellent sources of healthy fats that can aid in the assimilation of Vitamin D3. This practice not only maximizes the vitamin's efficacy but also makes it easier to form a habit when paired with regular meals.

Strategies for Maintaining Consistency

Consistency is key to effective supplementation. Here are some strategies to help maintain a regular routine:

1. *Set Reminders*

Utilize smartphone alarms or calendar notifications to remind you to take your supplement at the same time each day. Establishing a consistent routine not only helps you remember to take your supplement but also ensures that your body receives it at optimal intervals for the best results.

You can customize your reminders with specific labels, such as "Time for my vitamins!" to make them more engaging. Additionally, consider setting multiple reminders throughout the day, especially if you often find yourself getting distracted by daily tasks or commitments. This way, you'll have a gentle nudge to keep you on track and prioritize your health.

2. *Keep Supplements Visible*

One effective strategy for remembering to take your Vitamin D3 is to place the bottle in a prominent and frequently used spot within your home. Consider setting it next to your coffee maker, where you prepare your morning brew, on the dining table where you enjoy your meals, or near your toothbrush in the bathroom.

By ensuring that it's in your line of sight, you create a visual cue that nudges you to take your supplement regularly. This simple adjustment helps integrate the habit into your daily routine, making it easier to prioritize your health without adding extra steps to your day. Additionally, you might even consider pairing it with another daily activity, like enjoying your morning coffee or brushing your teeth, to further reinforce the habit.

3. **Link to an Established Habit**

    Pairing your supplement intake with an existing daily habit can be an effective strategy for ensuring consistency. For example, you might consider taking your supplements while enjoying your morning coffee, brushing your teeth, or sitting down for breakfast. This technique, known as habit stacking, takes advantage of the natural rhythm of your daily routine.

    By linking the act of taking supplements to a well-established habit, you create a mental cue that reminds you to take your supplements without having to consciously think about it. Over time, this can help you build a reliable routine that supports your health and wellness goals, making it easier to integrate supplements into your lifestyle seamlessly.

4. **Use a Pill Organizer**

    A weekly pill organizer is a crucial tool that can greatly assist in managing your daily doses, ensuring you never miss a day. By arranging your supplements by day and time, you can easily verify whether you've taken your dose, which is particularly advantageous if you take several supplements throughout the day.

This visual organization helps avoid confusion and the potential for missed doses, which can disrupt your health routine. Additionally, a well-structured pill organizer can serve as a reminder to maintain consistency in your health regimen, promoting better adherence to your wellness goals. Overall, it's a simple yet highly effective way to maintain your health and ensure that you are getting the most out of your supplements.

Incorporating Vitamin D3 into your daily routine requires a combination of choosing the right time, taking it with meals containing healthy fats, and employing strategies to maintain consistency. By adopting these practices, you can optimize the benefits of Vitamin D3 supplementation and support your ongoing health journey.

Step 5: Monitor Your Progress and Adjust as Needed

Once you have started your Vitamin D3 supplementation, it is essential to monitor your progress to ensure that your regimen is effective and safe. Regular check-ups and adjustments are crucial for maintaining optimal health and achieving the full benefits of supplementation.

The Importance of Regular Check-Ups

Scheduling regular check-ups with your healthcare provider is a critical step in effectively managing your Vitamin D3 supplementation. These appointments provide a valuable opportunity to review your Vitamin D levels through comprehensive blood tests, which allow for a precise assessment of your current status and overall health.

Regular monitoring is essential, as it helps in identifying any potential deficiencies or excesses early on, thereby minimizing health risks and optimizing positive outcomes. Vitamin D is vital for numerous body functions, such as maintaining bone health, supporting the body's immune system, and regulating mood.. By staying informed about your Vitamin D levels, you can make informed decisions about your supplementation and lifestyle choices.

Additionally, these check-ups facilitate open communication with your healthcare provider, allowing for personalized recommendations that take into account your unique health needs, lifestyle factors, and any other supplements or medications you may be taking. Prioritizing regular check-ups not only empowers you to take charge of your health but also fosters a proactive approach to maintaining your well-being in the long run.

Interpreting Vitamin D Level Results

Understanding your Vitamin D level results is vital for managing your supplementation effectively. Generally, Vitamin D levels are measured in nanograms per milliliter (ng/mL). A level between 20-50 ng/mL is typically considered adequate for most people.

Levels below 20 ng/mL may indicate a deficiency, while levels above 50 ng/mL could suggest excess and potential toxicity. Discussing these results with your healthcare provider will help you understand what they mean for your health and how they should influence your supplementation strategy.

Signs That Dosage Adjustments Might Be Necessary

Several signs could indicate the need for dosage adjustments:

- *Persistent Deficiency Symptoms:* If you continue to experience symptoms such as fatigue, bone pain, or muscle weakness despite taking Vitamin D supplements, it might be necessary to reassess your dosage. This ongoing discomfort could indicate that your current intake isn't sufficient to meet your body's needs, and consulting with a healthcare professional can help determine whether you need a higher dose or a different form of supplementation.

- *Changes in Lifestyle or Health Status:* Various factors, such as spending more time indoors due to seasonal changes, dietary adjustments that lower your intake of Vitamin D-rich foods, or the onset of new health conditions like obesity or gastrointestinal disorders, can significantly impact your Vitamin D requirements. It's essential to regularly evaluate your lifestyle and health status to ensure that your Vitamin D levels remain adequate for optimal health.

- ***Fluctuating Blood Levels:*** Regular testing that reveals inconsistent Vitamin D levels may necessitate dosage changes to stabilize and maintain optimal levels. These fluctuations can be influenced by several factors, including seasonal variations in sunlight exposure and changes in your body's absorption rates. Working with a healthcare provider to interpret these results can help tailor a supplementation plan that ensures you achieve and sustain healthy Vitamin D levels over time.

The Role of Healthcare Providers in Managing Supplementation

Healthcare providers play an indispensable role in guiding your Vitamin D3 supplementation journey. They can interpret blood test results, recommend appropriate dosage adjustments, and provide personalized advice based on your overall health and lifestyle. By maintaining open communication with your healthcare provider, you can ensure that your supplementation plan remains effective and tailored to your needs.

Monitoring your progress and making necessary adjustments are vital components of a successful Vitamin D3 supplementation regimen. Regular check-ups, understanding your Vitamin D levels, recognizing signs that adjustments are needed, and working closely with healthcare providers will help you achieve the best possible health outcomes through informed and effective supplementation.

By following these steps, you can safely and effectively incorporate Vitamin D3 supplements into your daily routine. Consistent supplementation can lead to improved bone health, enhanced immune function, and better mood regulation. Always consult with a healthcare professional to tailor your Vitamin D3 intake to your specific needs, ensuring optimal health benefits.

Precautions When Taking Vitamin D3 Supplements

When incorporating Vitamin D3 supplements into your health regimen, it's important to be aware of certain precautions to ensure safe and effective use. Here are key considerations to keep in mind:

1. **Potential Side Effects**

    While Vitamin D3 is typically safe for most individuals, but consuming too much can cause side effects like nausea, vomiting, constipation, and weakness. In severe cases, high levels of Vitamin D can result in hypercalcemia, a condition characterized by elevated calcium levels in the blood, which can cause kidney stones, bone pain, and cardiovascular issues.

2. **Interactions with Medications**

   Vitamin D3 can interact with various medications, potentially affecting their efficacy or leading to adverse effects. For instance, corticosteroids, weight loss drugs, and cholesterol-lowering medications may interfere with Vitamin D metabolism.

   Additionally, certain medications for heart conditions or epilepsy can be influenced by Vitamin D levels. Always consult with your healthcare provider or pharmacist about possible interactions if you are on any long-term medication.

3. **Risk of Over-Supplementation**

   Over-supplementation of Vitamin D3 can lead to toxicity, especially when taken in high doses over extended periods. This condition, known as Vitamin D toxicity, can cause calcium buildup in the blood, resulting in nausea, frequent urination, and even kidney damage. It is crucial to adhere to recommended dosages and have your levels monitored regularly by a healthcare professional.

4. Specific Health Conditions

Certain health conditions may require special attention when taking Vitamin D3 supplements:

- ***Kidney Disease***

  Individuals diagnosed with kidney disease often require adjusted dosages of Vitamin D, as their kidneys may struggle to convert this vitamin into its active form efficiently. This can lead to a deficiency, which is critical to address since Vitamin D plays a crucial role in maintaining bone health and regulating calcium levels in the body.

- ***Hyperparathyroidism***

  When hyperparathyroidism occurs, the parathyroid glands become excessively active, leading to an overproduction of parathyroid hormone (PTH). This excess can result in significantly high calcium levels in the bloodstream, a condition called hypercalcemia. This can trigger various health complications, such as kidney stones, bone discomfort, and digestive issues.

  In such situations, supplementing with Vitamin D may exacerbate hypercalcemia because

Vitamin D increases calcium absorption in the intestines. This can create further complications, particularly for individuals already struggling with elevated calcium levels.

It's essential for patients with hyperparathyroidism to monitor their Vitamin D intake closely and maintain open communication with their healthcare provider. Regular check-ups and tailored advice can help manage their condition effectively and ensure that any supplementation is appropriate and safe.

- *Cancer*

    Certain cancer treatments, such as chemotherapy and radiation, can significantly impact Vitamin D metabolism, potentially altering how the body absorbs and utilizes this essential vitamin. Vitamin D plays a crucial role in numerous bodily functions, including immune response, bone health, and cellular growth. Due to the complex nature of cancer therapies, it is critical for cancer patients to coordinate closely with their healthcare provider regarding Vitamin D supplementation.

This collaboration ensures that any supplementation does not interfere with their treatment plan or overall health. Additionally, healthcare providers can offer tailored advice on appropriate dosages and the best forms of Vitamin D to support the patient's unique needs during their cancer journey.

- ***Pregnancy and Breastfeeding***

    For pregnant or breastfeeding women, Vitamin D needs can significantly differ from those of the general population due to the vitamin's vital role in fetal development and infant health. It is crucial for these women to discuss their Vitamin D levels with their healthcare provider, who can recommend appropriate supplementation to support both their health and the health of their baby. Nutritional needs during this period might vary based on diet, sun exposure, and individual health factors.

Taking Vitamin D3 supplements can provide numerous health benefits, but it's important to do so safely. By understanding potential side effects, being aware of interactions with medications, avoiding over-supplementation, and considering specific health conditions, you can effectively incorporate Vitamin D3 into your health routine. Always consult with healthcare professionals for personalized advice and regular monitoring to ensure optimal results.

Potential Side Effects

While Vitamin D3 is generally safe for most individuals, it's important to be aware of potential side effects that can arise, especially with excessive intake. Understanding these effects can help you mitigate them effectively.

1. **Nausea and Vomiting**

   Nausea and vomiting are common side effects associated with excessive Vitamin D3 intake. This occurs because the body may struggle to process high levels of Vitamin D, which can disrupt normal digestive functions. To mitigate these symptoms, ensure that you are following the recommended dosage and consider taking the supplement with food to ease digestion.

2. **Constipation**

   Constipation can result from high levels of calcium in the blood triggered by excessive Vitamin D3 intake. This side effect is related to the role of Vitamin D in calcium absorption, where too much calcium can slow down bowel movements. To alleviate this, maintain adequate hydration, consume a fiber-rich diet, and monitor your Vitamin D intake to ensure it remains within safe limits.

3. **Weakness**

   Feelings of weakness or fatigue may occur due to an imbalance in mineral levels caused by high Vitamin D3 intake. Excessive Vitamin D can lead to an overabundance of calcium in the bloodstream, affecting muscle and nerve function. To prevent this, adhere to the recommended dosage and consult with a healthcare provider if you experience persistent weakness.

4. **Hypercalcemia**

   Hypercalcemia is a serious condition characterized by elevated calcium levels in the blood, which can result from excessive Vitamin D3 consumption. Symptoms of hypercalcemia include kidney stones, bone pain, and cardiovascular issues. This condition requires prompt medical attention. To avoid hypercalcemia, ensure your Vitamin D3 intake is within the recommended range and have your calcium levels monitored regularly by a healthcare professional.

While Vitamin D3 supplements offer numerous health benefits, being aware of potential side effects is crucial for safe usage. By understanding these effects and taking steps to mitigate them, you can effectively incorporate Vitamin D3 into your health regimen. Always consult with a healthcare provider to tailor your supplementation plan to your individual needs and ensure optimal health outcomes.

Tips for Maintaining Adequate Vitamin D3 Levels

Maintaining sufficient Vitamin D3 levels is crucial for overall health and well-being. Here are some practical tips to ensure you're getting enough of this vital nutrient:

Balancing Sunlight Exposure with Skin Protection

Optimal Sun Exposure

Achieving optimal sun exposure for Vitamin D3 synthesis involves a careful balance of time spent in the sun, taking into account several important factors like skin type, geographic location, and seasonal changes. Here's a detailed look at how to safely obtain the necessary sunlight:

1. ***Skin Type Considerations:*** Different skin types produce Vitamin D3 at different rates. Fair-skinned individuals typically need less sunlight exposure to produce the same amount of Vitamin D3 as those with darker skin, who may require more time outdoors. This

is due to higher melanin levels, which can reduce UVB absorption.

2. ***Geographic Location Influence:*** Your location plays a significant role in how much sunlight you receive. Those living closer to the equator can obtain Vitamin D3 more easily throughout the year due to consistent sunlight. In contrast, individuals in northern latitudes may experience reduced UVB radiation, particularly in winter months, necessitating longer exposure times or alternative sources like diet and supplements.

3. ***Seasonal Variations:*** During winter, the sun is lower in the sky, and its rays pass through more of the Earth's atmosphere, reducing UVB exposure. This can be compensated by spending more time outside when the sun is at its peak or by seeking alternatives on cloudy days.

4. ***Practical Sun Exposure Tips:*** To maximize Vitamin D3 production while protecting your skin, aim for short, frequent periods of sun exposure. Ideally, spend about 10 to 30 minutes in the midday sun, when UVB rays are most potent, between 10 AM and 3 PM. Adjust this time based on your personal and environmental factors, increasing exposure for darker skin tones or during overcast conditions.

5. ***Safety Measures:*** While pursuing sun exposure, protect your skin by applying sunscreen after initial exposure, wearing a hat, or using protective clothing if you plan to be outside longer than the recommended time. This helps prevent skin damage while allowing your body to produce adequate Vitamin D3.

By understanding and adjusting for these variables, you can effectively and safely harness the sun's rays to support your body's Vitamin D3 needs.

Mindful Skin Protection

Balancing sun exposure with mindful skin protection is crucial to safely obtain Vitamin D3 without risking skin damage. While sunlight is essential for Vitamin D3 synthesis, overexposure can lead to harmful effects like sunburn and increased skin cancer risk. Here's how to protect your skin while enjoying the sun's benefits:

1. ***Importance of Skin Protection:*** The sun's UV rays can cause both immediate and long-term skin damage. While short, unprotected sun exposure is beneficial for Vitamin D3 production, extended exposure without protection can lead to serious consequences, such as premature aging, hyperpigmentation, and skin cancer.

2. ***Choosing the Right Sunscreen:*** Choose a sunscreen that offers broad-spectrum protection with a minimum SPF of 30 to shield your skin from UVA and UVB

rays. Generously apply it to all exposed areas, such as your face and hands, after a brief period of unprotected exposure. Don't forget to reapply every after two hours, or more frequently if you're in the water or perspiring.

3. ***Role of Protective Clothing:*** To effectively protect your skin from excessive UV rays, consider wearing protective clothing. Choose long-sleeved tops, wide-brimmed hats, and sunglasses to shield vulnerable areas. Garments with a high Ultraviolet Protection Factor (UPF) provide enhanced defense.

4. ***Timing Your Sun Exposure:*** To minimize the risk of skin damage, plan your sun exposure when there's less UV radiation, usually outside of peak hours (10 AM to 3 PM). If you're outdoors during these times, seek shade or cover-up after your initial Vitamin D3-focused sun exposure.

5. ***Additional Tips for Mindful Exposure:*** Be aware of reflective surfaces like water, sand, and snow, which can intensify UV exposure. Use an SPF-infused lip balm to protect your lips, and avoid tanning beds, which can harm your skin without offering the Vitamin D3 benefits of natural sunlight.

By combining strategic sun exposure with effective skin protection, you are able to relish the health benefits of

Vitamin D3 while safeguarding the well-being and look of your skin.

Consider Your Location

Geographic location significantly impacts your ability to naturally produce Vitamin D3 from sunlight, particularly if you reside in northern latitudes or regions with limited sunshine. In these areas, the angle of the sun during winter months is lower, resulting in less UVB radiation reaching the Earth's surface. This can hinder your body's capacity to synthesize adequate Vitamin D3, necessitating alternative strategies to maintain healthy levels.

1. ***Understanding Geographic Impact:*** Those living further from the equator experience shorter days and less direct sunlight, especially during winter. This reduces the opportunity for effective Vitamin D3 production. As a result, residents of these areas need to be more proactive in compensating for this natural deficiency.

2. ***Dietary Adjustments:*** Incorporating more Vitamin D3-rich foods into your diet becomes crucial. Focus on consuming fatty fish like salmon and mackerel, fortified foods such as milk and cereals, and egg yolks. These sources can help bridge the gap left by inadequate sun exposure.

3. ***Supplementation Needs:*** Using Vitamin D3 supplements can be a practical solution, particularly during months when outdoor sunlight is insufficient for natural synthesis. Consult with a healthcare provider to determine the appropriate supplement dosage based on your specific needs and lifestyle.

4. ***Winter Strategies:*** During the colder months, when outdoor activity might be limited, it's essential to ensure your indoor diet compensates for the lack of sun exposure. Plan meals that are rich in Vitamin D3 and consider supplementing to maintain optimal health.

By understanding the influence of your location on Vitamin D3 production and making informed dietary and lifestyle choices, you can effectively support your body's needs regardless of the season or geographic constraints.

Time of Day Matters

The time of day plays a crucial role in optimizing Vitamin D3 production, primarily due to the sun's position in the sky. When the sun is at its highest point, typically between 10 AM and 3 PM, its rays are the most direct, providing the optimal conditions for UVB rays to penetrate the skin and stimulate Vitamin D3 synthesis effectively.

1. ***Impact of Sun Position:*** During these peak hours, the sun's UVB rays have the shortest path through the

atmosphere, minimizing absorption by air molecules and maximizing the amount reaching the Earth's surface. This makes it the most efficient time for your body to produce Vitamin D3.

2. *Optimizing Sun Exposure:* To harness these benefits, aim to spend about 10 to 30 minutes in the sun during these hours, depending on your skin type. Fair-skinned individuals often require less time to synthesize sufficient Vitamin D3 compared to those with darker skin, who may need more exposure due to higher melanin levels that can reduce UVB absorption.

3. *Safety Considerations:* It's important to balance sun exposure with skin protection to prevent potential damage. Limit your time in direct sunlight to the recommended duration and apply sunscreen afterward to protect your skin if you plan to stay outside longer. This helps prevent sunburn and reduces the risk of skin conditions.

4. *Adjustments for Skin Type:* Each skin type responds differently to UVB exposure. Darker skin tones should consider slightly extended exposure durations to achieve similar Vitamin D3 synthesis levels as lighter skin tones, while still taking care to avoid overexposure.

5. ***Practical Tips:*** If possible, schedule outdoor activities like walking or gardening during these peak hours to naturally boost your Vitamin D3 levels. Remember to stay hydrated and seek shade periodically to avoid overheating and excessive UV exposure.

By understanding the significance of the sun's position and adjusting your routine accordingly, you can effectively manage your Vitamin D3 levels while safeguarding your skin's health.

Incorporating Vitamin D3-rich Foods into the Diet

Incorporating Vitamin D3-rich foods into your diet is a strategic method to enhance your Vitamin D3 levels naturally. By prioritizing specific foods, you can ensure a steady intake of this essential nutrient, supporting your overall health.

1. ***Prioritize Fatty Fish:*** Fatty fish such as salmon, mackerel, tuna, and sardines are among the best natural sources of Vitamin D3. These fish are not only rich in Vitamin D3 but also provide heart-healthy omega-3 fatty acids. Aim to include servings of fatty fish in your diet at least twice a week. For instance, a dinner with grilled salmon or a tuna salad can significantly contribute to your Vitamin D3 intake.

2. ***Fortified Foods:*** Many everyday foods are fortified with Vitamin D3, making it easier to meet your nutritional needs. Look for fortified options like milk, orange juice, and breakfast cereals. When shopping, check food labels to ensure you're selecting products that add to your daily Vitamin D3 intake. A breakfast could feature fortified cereal with milk or a glass of fortified orange juice.

3. ***Egg Yolks and Cheese:*** Though containing smaller amounts of Vitamin D3 compared to fish, egg yolks and cheese can still play a valuable role in your diet. These foods are versatile and can be easily incorporated into meals. Consider adding eggs to your morning routine or including cheese as a snack or in salads.

4. ***Balanced Diet Planning:*** To integrate these Vitamin D3-rich foods naturally into your diet, plan meals that combine these sources. For example, start your day with a breakfast of scrambled eggs and fortified cereal, or enjoy a lunch featuring a salad with grilled salmon. Snacks like a cheese platter or fortified yogurt can further bolster your intake.

By incorporating a variety of these foods into your daily meals, you can effectively enhance your Vitamin D3 levels, promoting bone health, immune function, and overall well-being.

Choosing and Using Supplements Correctly

Choosing and using Vitamin D3 supplements correctly is an essential aspect of maintaining optimal health, particularly when natural sunlight exposure and dietary intake might not suffice. Here's a detailed guide to ensuring you manage your Vitamin D3 supplementation effectively and safely:

1. **Consult Healthcare Providers**

   Before starting any supplement regimen, it's crucial to have a discussion with your healthcare provider. They can help determine the appropriate dosage based on factors such as your current Vitamin D3 levels, dietary habits, lifestyle, and overall health status. This personalized approach ensures that you meet your nutritional needs without exceeding safe limits.

2. **Look for Quality Brands**

   When selecting Vitamin D3 supplements, opting for high-quality brands is essential to ensure you receive effective and safe products. Here's how you can navigate the supplement market to make informed choices:

   - ***Importance of Choosing High-Quality Supplements:*** Quality supplements guarantee that you're ingesting pure and potent forms of Vitamin D3 without unwanted additives or contaminants. High-quality supplements are more likely to deliver the health benefits you seek, such as improved bone health and immune function, and can help avoid potential side effects associated with lower quality products.

- ***Role of Third-Party Testing:*** Third-party testing is a critical factor in confirming the quality of supplements. These independent organizations test products for purity, potency, and safety, ensuring they contain what the label claims without harmful impurities. Look for supplements that explicitly mention third-party testing on their packaging or website, as this transparency indicates a commitment to quality.

- ***Identifying Certifications or Endorsements:*** Certifications from recognized health organizations can provide additional assurance of a supplement's quality. Look for seals from reputable entities such as the U.S. Pharmacopeia (USP), NSF International, or ConsumerLab. These endorsements indicate that the product has met stringent testing criteria, verifying its composition and effectiveness.

Practical Tips for Evaluating Supplement Brands:

- *Research Brands:* Start by researching brands with a solid reputation in the supplement industry. Look for customer reviews and feedback, which can give insights into product effectiveness and company reliability.

- *Check Labels:* Read product labels carefully to ensure transparency regarding ingredients and manufacturing processes. Avoid supplements with vague or incomplete labeling.

- *Consult Professionals:* Consider seeking advice from healthcare professionals or registered dietitians who can recommend reputable brands based on your health needs.

- *Making Informed Purchasing Decisions:* With numerous options available, prioritize brands that demonstrate quality control measures and transparency. Opt for products with clear labeling, verified by third-party testing, and endorsed by reputable health organizations. This approach will help you select supplements that support your health goals safely and effectively.

By paying attention to these factors, you can confidently choose Vitamin D3 supplements that provide the benefits you need while minimizing risks, ensuring your health and well-being are well-supported.

By following these tips, you can effectively balance sunlight exposure, incorporate Vitamin D3-rich foods, and choose supplements wisely to maintain adequate Vitamin D3 levels, supporting your bone health, immune function, and overall vitality.

Conclusion

As you reach the end of this comprehensive guide on Vitamin D3, let's take a moment to reflect on the journey and insights you've gained. Thank you for dedicating your time to learning about this vital nutrient. Your commitment to understanding Vitamin D3's role in your health is a commendable step towards enhancing your well-being.

Vitamin D3, often called the "sunshine vitamin," plays an integral role in various bodily functions. You've discovered that it's not just about supporting bone health, though that's a significant benefit. By aiding calcium absorption, Vitamin D3 ensures that your bones remain strong and resilient throughout your life. This is especially crucial as you age, helping to prevent conditions like osteoporosis.

But Vitamin D3's benefits extend beyond just bones. You've learned how it bolsters your immune system, acting as a crucial line of defense against infections and diseases. By maintaining optimal Vitamin D3 levels, you empower your body to fend off illnesses more effectively. This is particularly important in today's world, where maintaining robust health is a priority for many.

Additionally, you've seen how Vitamin D3 influences mood regulation. By participating in the production of neurotransmitters like serotonin, it helps in stabilizing mood and warding off depression. If you've ever experienced those winter blues, understanding and managing your Vitamin D3 levels could be part of the solution.

The guide has also highlighted the importance of getting your Vitamin D3 levels checked regularly. Since various factors—like age, skin color, geographical location, and dietary habits—can affect Vitamin D3 synthesis and absorption, it's crucial to have a personalized health strategy. Consulting with healthcare professionals allows you to tailor your Vitamin D3 intake to your specific needs, ensuring you're neither deficient nor consuming too much.

Moreover, you've explored natural ways to boost your Vitamin D3 levels. Simple lifestyle changes, such as spending more time in the sunlight, can significantly impact your Vitamin D3 synthesis. Sun exposure, in moderation, is one of the most effective ways to ensure your body gets adequate levels of this vitamin. However, remembering to maintain a balance in shielding your skin from harmful UV rays is essential for maintaining its health.

The diet also plays a pivotal role. Incorporating foods rich in Vitamin D3, such as fatty fish, fortified dairy products, and egg yolks, can be a delicious way to enhance your intake. Supplements are another viable option, especially if natural sources are insufficient or inaccessible due to lifestyle or geographical constraints.

Your newfound knowledge empowers you to make informed decisions about your health. You can now approach your diet and lifestyle with a clearer understanding of how to maintain optimal Vitamin D3 levels. This knowledge not only benefits you but can also be shared with loved ones, extending its positive impact.

As you move forward, keep the insights from this guide at the forefront of your wellness journey. Remember, maintaining healthy Vitamin D3 levels is not a one-time task but an ongoing commitment. Regular check-ups, a balanced diet, and mindful lifestyle choices go a long way in supporting your overall health.

Embrace this newfound understanding of Vitamin D3 as a tool to enhance your life quality. Whether it's strengthening your bones, boosting your immunity, or lifting your mood, you're now equipped to harness the full potential of this essential nutrient.

We encourage you to take your knowledge and put it into action. Monitor your Vitamin D3 levels, consult with healthcare providers, and make the necessary lifestyle changes to ensure you're living your healthiest life. Your health is a priority, and with this guide, you're well on your way to optimizing it.

FAQs

What is Vitamin D3, and why is it important for our health?

Cholecalciferol, commonly referred to as Vitamin D3, is an essential type of Vitamin D that plays a vital role in keeping bones and teeth healthy, bolstering the body's immune system, and ensuring muscles function correctly. It aids the body in absorbing calcium & phosphorus, which are critical for bone strength.

Where can Vitamin D3 be naturally sourced from?

Vitamin D3 is primarily synthesized in the skin through exposure to sunlight. Additionally, it can be found in certain foods, including fish liver oils, fortified cereals and milk, egg yolks, as well as fatty fish such as salmon and mackerel.

What is the recommended daily dosage of Vitamin D3?

The suggested daily amount of Vitamin D3 differs based on gender, age, and life stage. Typically, adults should aim for 600 to 800 IU per day. However, individual requirements can vary, so it's advisable to seek personalized advice from a healthcare professional.

What are the signs of Vitamin D3 deficiency?

Common signs of Vitamin D3 deficiency include fatigue, bone pain, muscle weakness, mood changes, and increased susceptibility to infections. Chronic deficiency can lead to more serious health issues such as osteoporosis or rickets in children.

Are there any potential side effects of taking Vitamin D3 supplements?

While Vitamin D3 is generally safe when taken in recommended doses, excessive intake can lead to toxicity, with symptoms such as nausea, vomiting, weakness, and serious complications like kidney damage. It's important to adhere to the recommended dosage and consult with a healthcare professional.

How can I choose the right Vitamin D3 supplement?

When selecting a Vitamin D3 supplement, consider factors such as the dosage, form (e.g., liquid, capsule, tablet), brand reputation, and additional ingredients. Look for products that have been third-party tested for quality and purity.

What is the best time to take Vitamin D3 supplements?

Vitamin D3 supplements are best absorbed when taken with a meal containing fats, as it is a fat-soluble vitamin. Consistency is key, so try to take it at the same time each day to help maintain adequate levels in your body.

References and Helpful Links

Stines, Y. (2024, August 15). Vitamin D3 benefits for glowing skin, heart health, and more. Verywell Health.
https://www.verywellhealth.com/vitamin-d3-5082500

National Library of Medicine. (n.d.). Vitamin D deficiency.
https://medlineplus.gov/vitaminddeficiency.html#:~:text=Vitamin%20D%20deficiency%20can%20lead,to%20become%20soft%20and%20bend.

Gurova, D. (2024, September 5). How to choose Vitamin D3: dosing, levels, form, and route of administration. Maxler.
https://maxler.com/blog/how-to-choose-vitamin-d3-dosing-levels-form-and-route-of-administration/

WebMD Editorial Contributor. (2022b, November 24). Foods high in vitamin D3. WebMD.
https://www.webmd.com/diet/foods-high-in-vitamin-d3

Vitamin D3 oral: Uses, side effects, interactions, pictures, warnings & dosing - WebMD. (n.d.).
https://www.webmd.com/drugs/2/drug-10175/vitamin-d3-oral/details#:~:text=Too%20much%20vitamin%20D%20can,%2Fmood%20changes%2C%20unusual%20tiredness.

Ajmera, R. (2024, January 5). Vitamin D3: benefits, sources, deficiency and risks. Forbes Health.
https://www.forbes.com/health/supplements/vitamin-d3/#:~:text=%E2%

80%9CVitamin%20D3%20is%20essential%20for,nutrition%20practice%20in%20Elkhorn%2C%20Wisconsin.

Made, N. (2023, May 9). When to take vitamin D: morning or night? Nature Made®. https://www.naturemade.com/blogs/health-articles/when-to-take-vitamin-d-morning-or-night#:~:text=While%20Vitamin%20D%20can%20be,in%20the%20evening%20before%20bed.